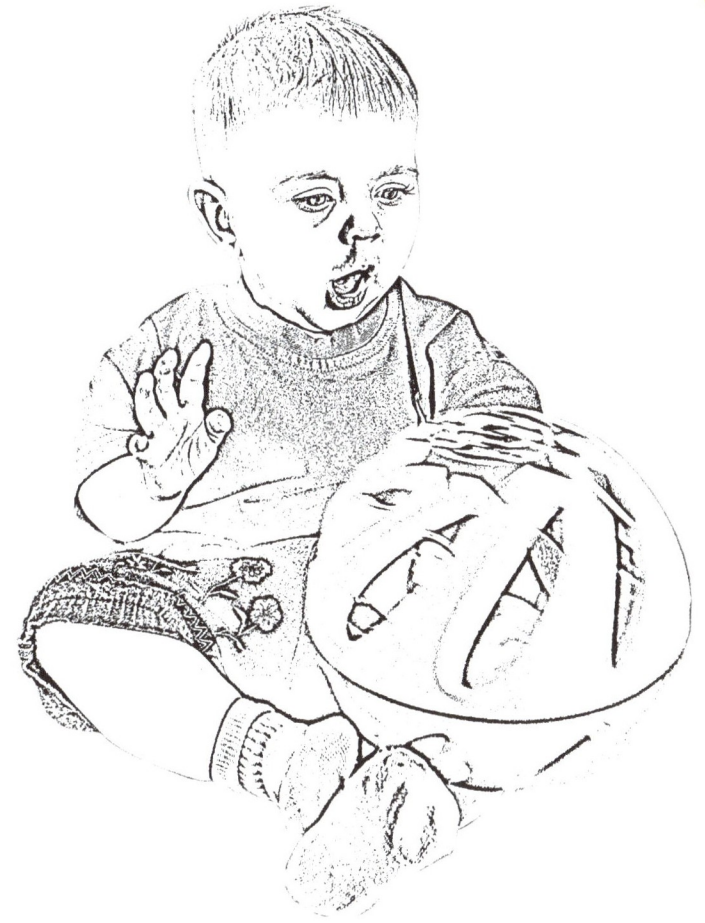

Milestones & Memories
Baby Record Book and Beyond

Your Child's Name _____

Birthdate _____

Written and designed by Barbara A. Fanson
Published by Sterling Education Centre Inc.

You can order additional forms or books on our website:
www.Fanson.net

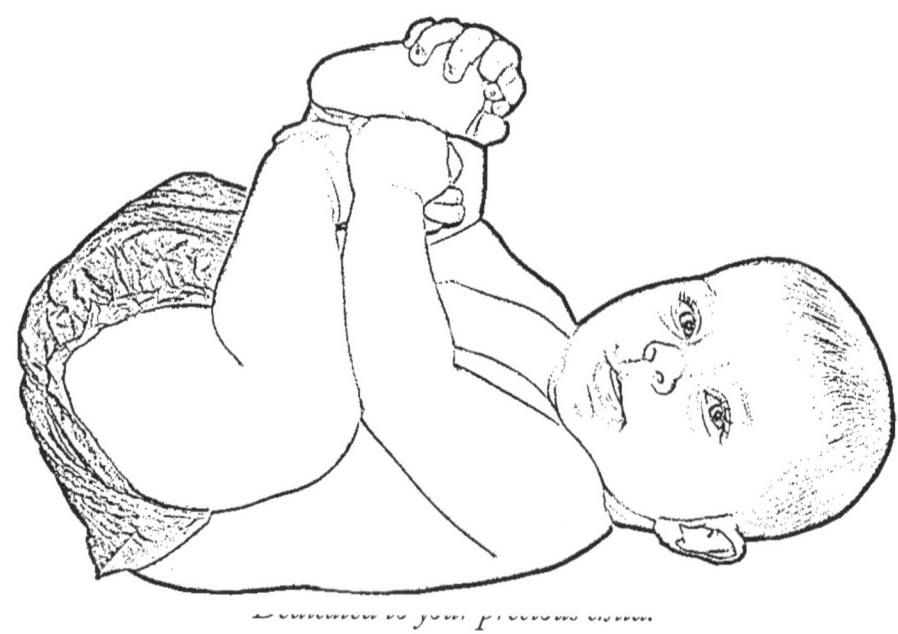

Copyright © 2016 Barbara A. Fanson

Written, illustrated, and designed by Barbara A. Fanson

All rights reserved.

Amazon: ISBN 9780993996344
Electronic ISBN: 978-1-989361-08-5
Ingram ISBN: 978-1-989361-09-2

13 pt. Adobe Caslon Pro on 18 pt leading.

No part of this publication may be reproduced or stored in a retrieval system, or transmitted in any form or by any means, electronic, mechanical, recording, or otherwise, without written permission of the publisher,

Sterling Education Centre Inc.
220 Homebrook Drive, Mount Hope, ON L0R 1W0
Email: Barbara@Fanson.net
www.Fanson.net
Telephone: (905) 679-9229

In the case of photocopying or other reprographic copying,
a license must be obtained from Sterling Education Centre Inc.

Contents

Preface	4
Your Pregnancy or Adoption	5
Your Baby's Birth	6
How Baby Has Grown	7
Baby's Handprints and Footprints	8
My Baby's Name	9
Where was I when labor started	10
Hospital Visitors	11
Baby Showers	12
What to bring to the hospital	13
The baby's list of what to bring	14
Equipping the nursery	15
Baby's Visitors	16, 17
Baby's Gifts	18
Baptism or Christening	19
Your Child's Growth	20
Planning Baby's First Birthday	21
Baby's First Birthday	22
Baby's Milestones, Dates	23, 24
Medical Visits	25 – 27
Measurements	28, 29
Immunization Schedule	30 – 32
Baby's First Teeth	33
Erupting Baby's First Teeth	34
Baby's First Teeth	35
Shedding Baby's First Teeth	36
Dental Visits	37, 38
Orthodontist Visits	39, 40
Certificates and Awards	41
Events and Activities	42
Baby's First Days	43 – 46
Memories of Pre-School	47
Memories of Kindergarten	48
Memories of Grade 1	49 – 56
Memories of Grade 9	57 – 60
Memories: Post-Secondary School	61
Jobs	62
Awards and Certificates	63
Observations and Comments	64

Preface

After miscarrying my first two pregnancies, I was anxious about this baby growing inside me. Anxious, but excited, and scared. She was ten days late, which gave me time to create my own Baby Record Book. It has evolved over the years, but I still use the original copy to document my precious gift. And now, it is ready to share with your little one.

Use this book to keep track of vaccinations, doctor appointments, and dentists. Use *Milestones & Memories* to record significant moments like how you first found out you were pregnant, baby showers, gifts, the birth, visitors, and milestones.

Moments, milestones, and memories preserved for your little one.

If you run out of forms or need another book, please visit our website: www.Fanson.net

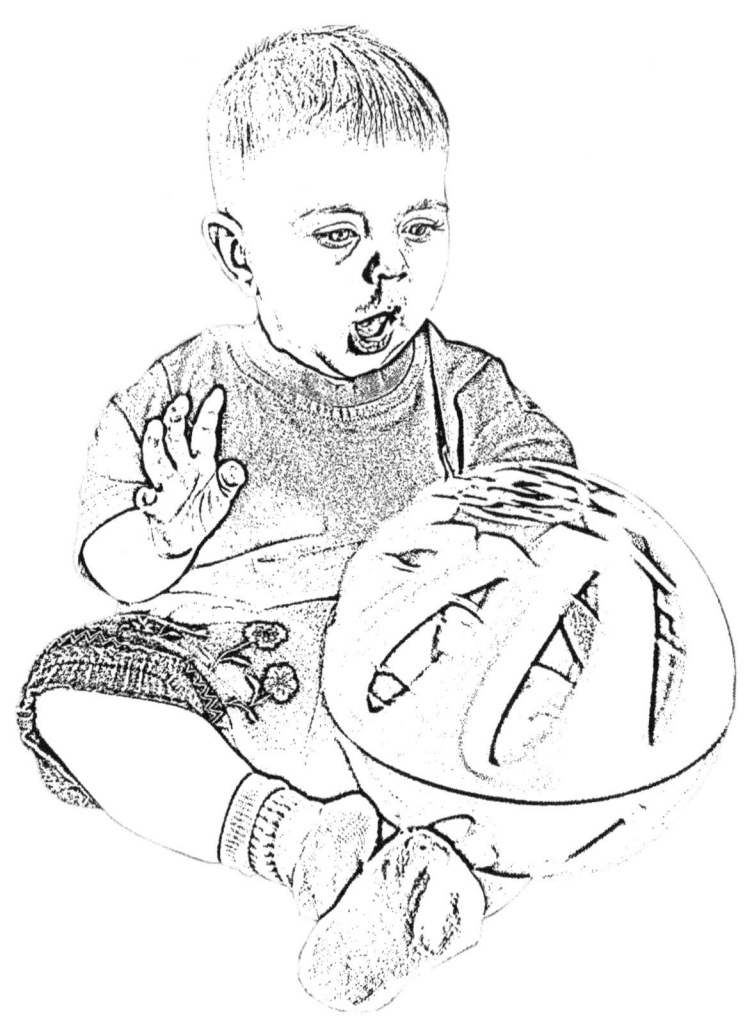

Your Pregnancy or Adoption

Record your thoughts and reactions when you found out you were pregnant or going to adopt.

Date _____

How _____

Where _____

My thoughts _____

_____

_____

_____

_____

_____

_____

_____

_____

_____

_____

_____

_____

_____

_____

_____

_____

Your Baby's Birth

Record details of your child's birth.

Date _____

Time _____

Weight _____

Where _____

City _____

Doctor or Midwife _____

Hair Color _____

Eye Color _____

Additional notes _____

_____

_____

_____

_____

_____

_____

_____

_____

_____

_____

_____

_____

How Baby Has Grown

Record your child's height and weight each year on their birthday or first day of school.

Age	Weight	Height
Birth		
Hospital discharge		
One month		
Two months		
Three months		
Four months		
Five months		
Six months		
Seven months		
Eight months		
Nine months		
Ten months		
Eleven months		
One Year		
Eighteen months		
Twenty-one months		
Two Years		

Age	Weight	Height

Baby Record Book

Baby's Handprints and Footprints

Paint one of your child's hands and a foot and press on this page. Or, use a large stamp pad.

My Baby's Name

How did you come up with your child's name?

Baby's full name _____

_____

Meaning and origin of Baby's name _____

_____

_____

_____

_____

Other names we considered _____

_____

_____

_____

_____

Baby's nicknames _____

_____

_____

_____

_____

Additional comments _____

_____

_____

_____

_____

Where was I when labor started

Record the date and time you went into labor and your symptoms.

Date _____

Where _____

Time _____

First Symptom _____

_____

Second Symptom _____

_____

Was anyone else present? _____

_____

Your reaction _____

_____

_____

_____

Where was Dad when you went into labor? _____

_____

_____

What time did you call the doctor or midwife? _____

What time did you leave for the hospital? _____

Did you tell anyone you were in labor? _____

Additional comments _____

_____

_____

Baby Record Book

Hospital Visitors

The following people visited us at the hospital or telephoned us. You can also record flowers received.

Baby Showers

Record any Baby Showers that were given for you before or after your child's birth. You can also record gifts.

Date _____

Given by _____

Place _____

City _____

Additional notes _____

_____

_____

_____

_____

_____

_____

_____

_____

_____

_____

_____

_____

_____

_____

What to bring to the hospital

Check off items as you pack your suitcase to take to the hospital.
You might want to have two suitcases: one for labor and one for your husband to bring later.

Labor Suitcase

- [ ] Health card
- [ ] proof of health insurance
- [ ] cord blood bank kit (if registered)
- [ ] long t-shirt or nightie
- [ ] robe
- [ ] socks or slippers
- [ ] sanitary napkins (hospital may supply)
- [ ] disposable underwear (Kotex)
- [ ] pillows
- [ ] popsicles or freezies
- [ ] lip balm or lip care (for dry lips)
- [ ] eyeglasses and container for contact lens
- [ ] mouth wash
- [ ] toothbrush and toothpaste
- [ ] hair brush
- [ ] hair tie or hair band
- [ ] shower cap
- [ ] moisturizer
- [ ] plastic covers (for your bed or furniture)
- [ ] music: iPad or CDs
- [ ] camera or video camera (battery charger)
- [ ] magazines, books, deck of cards
- [ ] comfort aids (rolling pin, tennis ball)
- [ ] massage oil or corn starch
- [ ] nourishment (jello, broth, herbal tea, clear juice, crackers, yogurt)
- [ ] small knit cap for baby (hospital supply?)
- [ ] swim suits (for mother and partner)
- [ ] birth plan
- [ ] ice packs
- [ ] _____

Postpartum Suitcase

- [ ] night gowns (open in front to breastfeed)
- [ ] robe
- [ ] slippers
- [ ] toiletries and cosmetics
- [ ] hair dryer and curling iron
- [ ] sanitary napkins (heavy)
- [ ] nursing bra
- [ ] breast pads
- [ ] clothes to wear home (you and baby)
- [ ] snacks (fruit, muffins)
- [ ] money (change for snack machine)
- [ ] credit card (for telephone, TV, photos)
- [ ] cell phone and charger
- [ ] contact list or address book
- [ ] car seat
- [ ] book and magazines
- [ ] notebook and pencil
- [ ] underwear or panties

For the birth partner

- [ ] watch with second hand
- [ ] food (sandwiches, fruit, crackers, cheese)
- [ ] fluids (juice, water, pop)
- [ ] change of clothes
- [ ] toiletries (toothbrush, razor, deodorant)
- [ ] swim suit (if needed)
- [ ] paper and pen
- [ ] contact list or list of phone numbers
- [ ] coins for snack machine
- [ ] Aspirin
- [ ] camera, video camera, and battery charger

The baby's list of what to bring to the hospital

Check off items as you pack the baby's suitcase to take to the hospital.
Some hospitals are not supplying as many baby items, as in the past.

First day at hospital

- ☐ socks
- ☐ booties
- ☐ receiving blankets
- ☐ disposable or cloth diapers
- ☐ small knitted cap
- ☐ spit up blankets
- ☐ bibs
- ☐ _____
- ☐ _____
- ☐ _____
- ☐ _____
- ☐ _____
- ☐ _____
- ☐ _____
- ☐ _____
- ☐ _____
- ☐ _____

Going home from hospital

- ☐ car seat
- ☐ undershirt
- ☐ diapers
- ☐ gown or sleeper
- ☐ booties or socks
- ☐ petroleum jelly
- ☐ facecloths or baby wipes
- ☐ hat
- ☐ mittens (depending on weather)
- ☐ coat (depending on weather)
- ☐ sweater
- ☐ bunting bag
- ☐ blanket
- ☐ _____
- ☐ _____
- ☐ _____
- ☐ _____
- ☐ _____
- ☐ _____
- ☐ _____

Equipping the nursery

Before you have your baby, you may want to make sure the nursery is ready and that you have enough items for baby's arrival.

Preparing the nursery

- [ ] crib or bassinet
- [ ] change table (any surface will do)
- [ ] bedding (2 fitted sheets and 1 blanket)
- [ ] waterproof pad or mattress pad
- [ ] bath supplies (baby tub or laundry basket in bathtub)
- [ ] hooded towel for bath
- [ ] wash cloths for face and behind
- [ ] mild laundry detergent (Ivory Snow?)
- [ ] baby thermometer
- [ ] undershirts (4 to 6)
- [ ] diapers (8 to 12 per day, minimum)
- [ ] night gowns (4 to 6)
- [ ] lighweight footed sleepers (summer)
- [ ] heavier footed sleepers (winter)
- [ ] socks (6 pairs)
- [ ] booties
- [ ] bibs (6)

receving blankets (3 to 5)

- [ ] outdoor clothing (depends on weather)
- [ ] blankets
- [ ] hat and mittens (1 or 2, depends on weather)
- [ ] _____
- [ ] _____
- [ ] _____
- [ ] _____
- [ ] _____
- [ ] _____

Toiletries

- [ ] brush and comb
- [ ] mild soap
- [ ] petroleum jelly
- [ ] baby powder
- [ ] baby nail scissors or clippers
- [ ] nasal bulb syringe
- [ ] baby shampoo
- [ ] diaper rash ointment
- [ ] baby oil
- [ ] baby wipes
- [ ] cotton balls
- [ ] rubbing alcohol
- [ ] _____
- [ ] _____
- [ ] _____

Diaper Bag

- [ ] diapers (4 to 6)
- [ ] bibs
- [ ] spare outfit
- [ ] pacifier
- [ ] formula
- [ ] couple of bottles
- [ ] baby wipes
- [ ] toys
- [ ] _____
- [ ] _____
- [ ] _____

Baby's Visitors

Use this page to record visitors after the birth of your baby.

Guest	City	Relationship	Comments

Baby's Visitors

Use this page to record visitors after the birth of your baby.

Guest	City	Relationship	Comments

Baby's Gifts

Use this page to record gifts your baby or you received.

Guest	Relationship	Thanks Sent	Gifts

Need more forms? Download them for free: www.Fanson.net

Baptism or Christening

Use this page to record information on your baby's baptism or christening.

Child's Full Name _____

Father's Name _____

Mother's Name _____

Date and Time _____

Church/Place of Worship _____

Address _____

Religious Leader _____

Godparent(s) _____

_____

_____

Other activities _____

_____

Guest	Relationship	Thanks Sent	Gifts

Your Child's Growth

At your child's regular check-ups, ask for the child's weight, height, and head size.

Date	Age	Weight	Length/Height	Head Size	Other

Need more forms? Download them for free: www.Fanson.net

Planning Baby's First Birthday

Use this page to plan activities for your baby's first birthday.

Activity _____

Theme _____

Date _____ Time _____

Place _____

Hosted by _____

Comments _____

_____

Who will you invite? (*List them on the next page.*) _____

_____

_____

☐ Videos
☐ Photo album

Party Decorations Theme
☐ Streamers   ☐ Banners
☐ Wall Decorations ☐ Table Decorations
☐ Party Plates   ☐ Party Cups _____
☐ Cutlery   ☐ Napkins _____

Balloons _____

_____

Loot Bags _____

Games/Activities _____

_____

_____

_____

_____

Prizes _____

_____

Birthday Cake _____

_____

_____

Refreshments _____

_____

_____

_____

Food _____

_____

_____

_____

_____

_____

_____

_____

_____

Baby's First Birthday

Use this page to record activities to celebrate baby's first birthday.

Activity _____

Theme _____

Date_____ Time _____

Comments_____

_____

Games/Activities_____

_____

_____

Name	Invite Sent	Thanks Sent	Gift

Baby's Milestones and Important Dates

Use this page to record important dates and "firsts" in your baby's life.

Date of birth _____ Time _____

Height _____ Weight _____

Apgar score _____ Date went home _____

First outing _____
_____

First health care providers visit _____

First bath _____

First haircut _____

First professional haircut _____

First holiday _____

First playmate _____

Smiles _____ Shakes a rattle _____

Lifts head _____ Holds a bottle _____

Laughs out loud _____ Drinks from a cup _____

Tracks a moving object _____ Sits alone _____

Discovers hands _____ Stands with support _____

Discovers feet _____ Sticks tongue out _____

Lays on floor _____ First cold _____

Bats at a toy _____ Creeping _____

Favorite toy _____ First kiss for Mommy _____

Reaches for an object _____ Pulls herself up _____

Sleeps through the night _____ Waves good-bye _____

Eats solid food _____ Claps hands _____

Favorite food _____ Rolls a ball _____

Says "da da" _____ Cuts a tooth _____

Says "ma" or "ga" _____ Crawls _____

Sits supported _____ Walks assisted _____

Rolls over _____ Stands alone _____

Baby Record Book

Baby's Milestones and Important Dates

Use this page to record more important dates and "firsts" in your baby's life.

Takes a step _____

Sits in a high chair _____

Other first words _____

_____

_____

_____

_____

Uses a spoon _____

Feeds self _____

Walks alone _____

Weight at first check-up (approx. 2 weeks)

_____

Height at first check-up _____

Puts foot in mouth _____

Others _____

Sits in first snow _____

First bandage _____

Blows bubbles in water _____

First pee-pee in potty _____

First poopoo in potty _____

First pee-pee in toilet _____

First poopoo in toilet _____

First vaccination _____

_____

First vacation _____

_____

Blows soapy bubbles _____

Drinks from regular glass _____

Drinks with straw _____

_____
_____
_____
_____
_____
_____
_____
_____
_____
_____
_____
_____
_____
_____

Baby Record Book

Medical Visits

Use this page to record visits to the doctor or health care provider. You can also record comments, immunizations, and prescriptions.

Date	Age	Weight	Height	Comments/Immunizations/Prescriptions

Medical Visits

Use this page to record visits to the doctor or health care provider. You can also record comments, immunizations, and prescriptions.

Date	Age	Weight	Height	Comments/Immunizations/Prescriptions

Medical Visits

Use this page to record visits to the doctor or health care provider. You can also record comments, immunizations, and prescriptions.

Date	Age	Weight	Height	Comments/Immunizations/Prescriptions

Need more forms? Download them for free: www.Fanson.net

Measurements

Use this page to record your child's height, weight, and measurements. You may want to measure a baby weekly, but once they turn 1 year, then measure on their birthday and first day of school.

Date	Age	Weight	Height	Date	Age	Weight	Height

Measurements

Use this page to record your child's height, weight, and measurements. You may want to measure a baby weekly, but once they turn 1 year, then measure on their birthday and first day of school.

Date	Age	Weight	Height	Date	Age	Weight	Height

Need forms? Download: www.Fanson.net

Immunization Schedule

This is a general guideline for infants and children which varies from province to province.

Age & Date at vaccination	DTap[1]	Inactivated polio vaccine	Hib[2]	MMR[3]	Td[4]	Hep B[5] (3 doses)
Birth						
2 months	X	X	X			
4 months	X	X	X			
6 months	X	X	X			
12 months				X		
18 months	X	X	X	X[6]		
4 – 6 years	X	X		X[6]		
14 – 16 years					X	

1. DTap — Diphtheria, tetanus, pertussis (acellular) vaccine.
2. Hib — Haemophilus influenza type b to conjugate vaccine.
3. MMR — Measles, mumps, rubella vaccine.
4. Td — Tetanus and diphtheria.
   A booster shot is recommended every 10 years.
5. Hep B — Hepatitis B vaccine.
   3 does: infancy or preadolescence (9 – 13 years)
6. A second dose of MMR is given at 18 months, or at the start of the school year, depending on where you live.

Immunization Record

Record vaccinations or immunizations. Please check with your doctor for vaccinations.

Vaccine	Date	Comment	Doctor
Hep B 1			
Hep B 2			
Hep B 3			
DTaP 1			
DTaP 2			
DTaP3			
DTaP4			
DTaP5			
Hib 1			
Hib 2			
Hib 3			
Polio 3			
Polio 4			
DT			
Td			
MMR 1			
MMR 2			
Varicella			
TB test			
HGB			

Need more forms? Download them for free: www.Fanson.net

Immunization Schedule

Record optional vaccinations or travel immunizations.

Date of vaccination	Age	Type of Immunization	Doctor

Need more forms? Download them for free: www.Fanson.net

Baby's First Teeth

Babies usually have 20 primary teeth which will start to erupt (show) at 6 to 10 months of age.

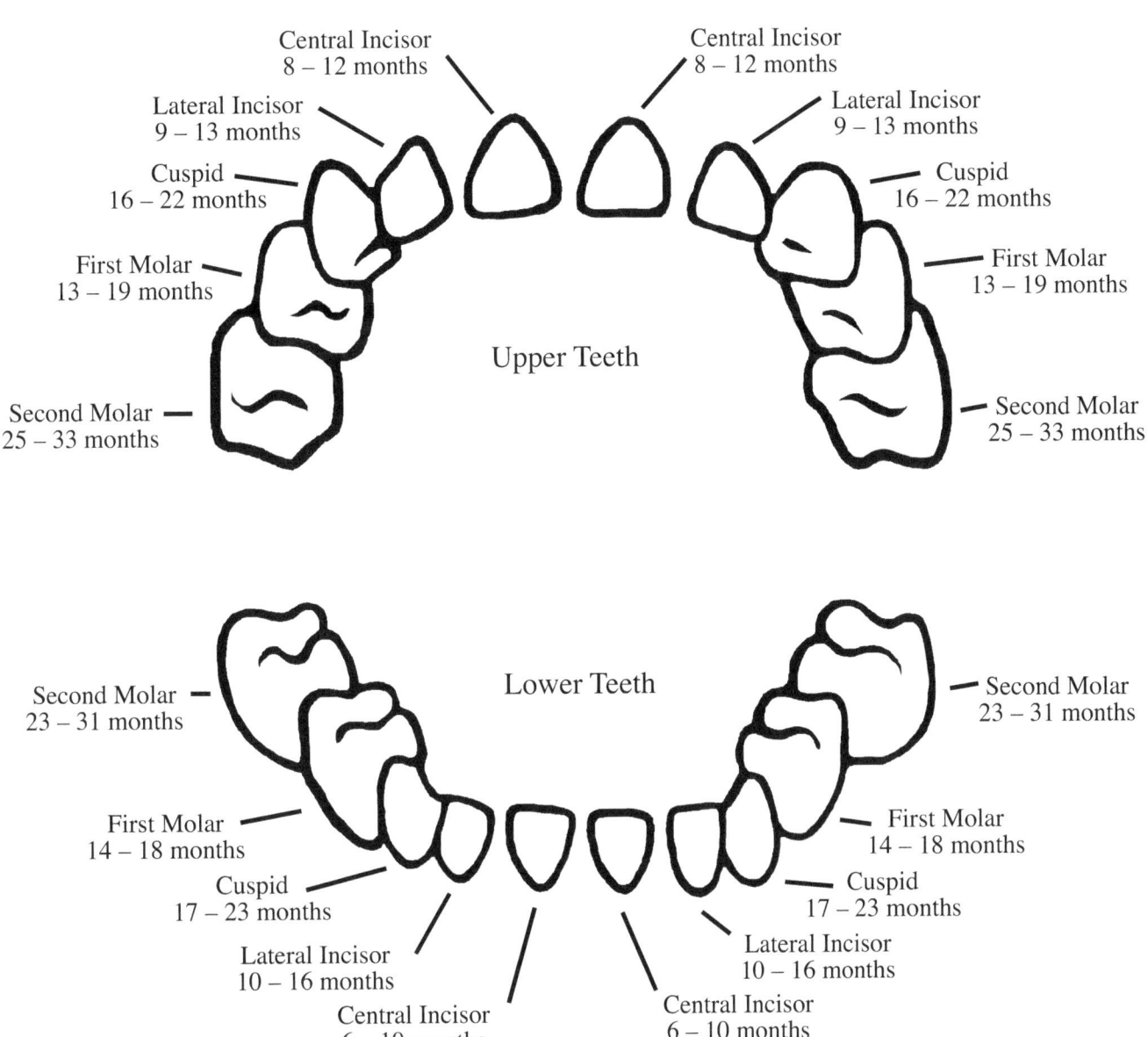

Erupting Baby's First Teeth

Use this chart to record eruption or showing of baby's first teeth.

L = Left R = Right		Eruption Average	Eruption Date	Age (yrs, months)
Upper Teeth				
Central Incisor	L	8 – 12 mos.		
	R	8 – 12 mos.		
Lateral Incisor	L	9 – 13 mos.		
	R	9 – 13 mos.		
Cuspid	L	16 – 22 mos.		
	R	16 – 22 mos.		
First Molar	L	13 – 19 mos.		
	R	13 – 19 mos.		
Second Molar	L	25 – 33 mos.		
	R	25 – 33 mos.		
Lower Teeth				
Central Incisor	L	8 – 12 mos.		
	R	8 – 12 mos.		
Lateral Incisor	L	9 – 13 mos.		
	R	9 – 13 mos.		
Cuspid	L	16 – 22 mos.		
	R	16 – 22 mos.		
First Molar	L	13 – 19 mos.		
	R	13 – 19 mos.		
Second Molar	L	25 – 33 mos.		
	R	25 – 33 mos.		

Need more forms? Download them for free: www.Fanson.net

Baby's First Teeth

Babies usually have 20 primary teeth which will start to erupt (show) at 6 to 10 months of age.

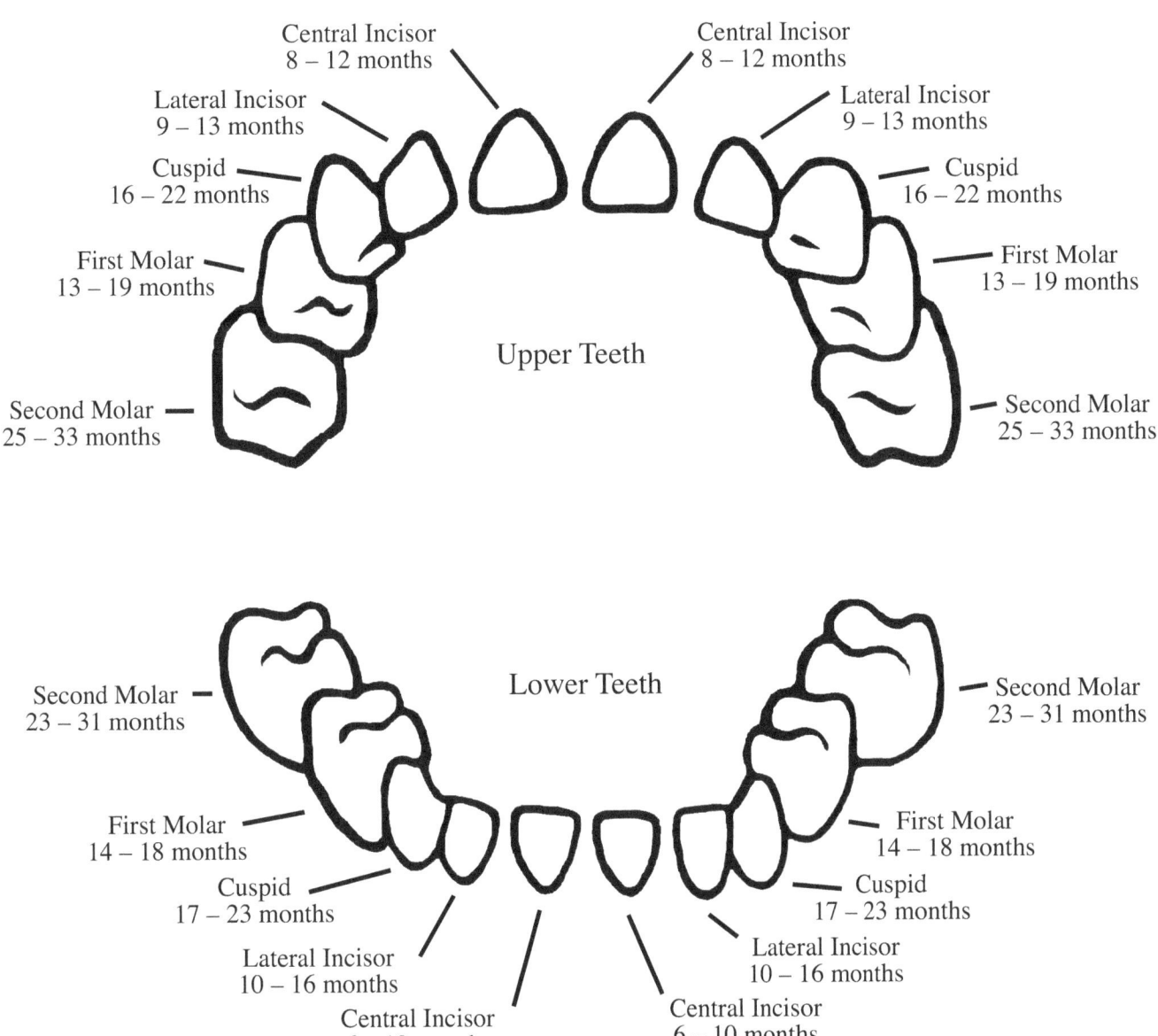

Baby Record Book   35

Shedding Baby's First Teeth

Use this chart to record shedding or losing of baby's first teeth.

L = Left R = Right		Shedding Average	Shedding Date	Age (yrs, months)
Upper Teeth				
Central Incisor	L	6 – 7 yrs.		
	R	6 – 7 yrs.		
Lateral Incisor	L	7 – 8 yrs.		
	R	7 – 8 yrs.		
Cuspid	L	10 – 12 yrs.		
	R	10 – 12 yrs.		
First Molar	L	9 – 11 yrs.		
	R	9 – 11 yrs.		
Second Molar	L	10 – 12 yrs.		
	R	10 – 12 yrs.		
Lower Teeth				
Central Incisor	L	6 – 7 yrs.		
	R	6 – 7 yrs.		
Lateral Incisor	L	7 – 8 yrs.		
	R	7 – 8 yrs.		
Cuspid	L	10 – 12 yrs.		
	R	10 – 12 yrs.		
First Molar	L	9 – 11 yrs.		
	R	9 – 11 yrs.		
Second Molar	L	10 – 12 yrs.		
	R	10 – 12 yrs.		

Need more forms? Download them for free: www.Fanson.net

Dental Visits

Record visits to a dentist and what service was performed. Most dentists recommend the first visit at 3 years of age.

Dentist's Name _____

Address _____

Telephone _____

Date of first tooth showing and child's age_____

Age when your child started brushing his/her teeth_____

Age and date of first visit to the dentist _____

Date	Age	Service

Dental Visits

Date	Age	Service

Need more forms? Download them for free: www.Fanson.net

Orthodontist Visits

Record visits to an orthodontist and what service should be performed.

Orthodontist's Name _____

Address _____

Telephone _____

Age and date of first visit to the orthodontist _____

Recommendations/Comments _____

_____

Date	Age	Service/Comment

Orthodontist Visits

Record visits to an orthodontist and what service should be performed.

Date	Age	Service

Need more forms? Download them for free: www.Fanson.net

Certificates and Awards

Record any certificates, awards, or prizes your child earns or wins.

Date	Organization	Certificate/Award/Prize

Need more forms? Download them for free: www.Fanson.net

Events and Activities

Use this page to record events, activities, or trips in your child's life.

Date	Where	Event or Activity

Need more forms? Download them for free: www.Fanson.net

Baby's First Days

You may nurse your baby an average of 8 to 12 times in the first 24 hours, or every 1.5 to 3 hours. The baby should appear content after nursing. These are

Day 1 to 3   Colostrum
                Bowel movements: 1 to 3 sticky, dark green to almost black.
                Wet diapers: generally 2 to 3, increasing the number and amount each day.

Day 3 to 4   Milk coming in
                Bowel movements: 3 to 4 brown/green/yellow in color.
                Wet diapers: 3 to 4 per day, heavier wetting.

Day 5 to 6   Mature milk
                Bowel movements: 3 to 5 or more, becoming more yellow in color.
                At least 3 are the size of a dollar coin.
                Heavy wet diapers: 5 to 7 per day.

If your baby is latched well:
- ✓ See ☛ Mouth open wide
- ✓ See ☛ Lips flanged out and relaxed
- ✓ Feel ☛ Breast tug—no pain
- ✓ See ☛ Slow rhythmic sucking
- ✓ Hear ☛ The sound of the baby swallowing

Call for help if:
- Nipples are sore or cracked
- Unable to get baby latched onto breast
- Baby has only rapid, nibbling, shallow type of sucking
- No bowel movements for over 12 hours in the first week
- Baby has dark green or black stools after Day 5
- Baby has infrequent wet diapers after Day 3
- Baby falls asleep after nursing for only a few minutes.
- Baby sleeps for 4 to 5 hours more than once a day.
- Baby is spending more than 45 minutes at the breast and begins crying soon after being taken off.
- Baby is not content between feeding, wails, or cries a lot.

Baby's First Days

Keeping this record will help you keep track of your baby's feedings and diaper changes during the first few days when are too busy and too tired to remember them. It will help you decide if your baby is getting enough to drink and will be helpful when visiting a midwife or doctor.

Day	Time	Length of Feed L Breast R	Urine	Stool	Stool Color	Comments
Mon.	7 a.m.	10 min.	no	✓	black, sticky	Not very interested
Wed.	9 a.m.	20 min.	✓	no		Sucked well

Need more forms? Download them for free: www.Fanson.net

Baby's First Days (Breastfed)

Keeping this record will help you keep track of your baby's feedings and diaper changes during the first few days when are too busy and too tired to remember them. It will help you decide if your baby is getting enough to drink and will be helpful when visiting a midwife or doctor.

Day	Time	Length of Feed L Breast R	Urine	Stool	Stool Color	Comments
Mon.	7 a.m.	10 min.	no	✓	black, sticky	Not very interested
Wed.	9 a.m.	20 min.	✓	no		Sucked well

Need more forms? Download them for free: www.Fanson.net

Baby's First Days (Bottle-fed)

Keeping this record will help you keep track of your baby's feedings and diaper changes during the first few days when are too busy and too tired to remember them. It will help you decide if your baby is getting enough to drink and will be helpful when visiting a midwife or doctor.

Day	Time	Feeding	Urine	Bowel	Comments
Mon.	7 a.m.	6 oz.	no	✓	She seems fine.

Need more forms? Download them for free: www.Fanson.net

Memories of Pre-School

Record some of your child's friends at home or pre-school or child care. Feel free to attach photos or other memorababilia. List the names of pre-schools or daycare facilities attended.

Memories of Kindergarten

Record some of your child's friends at home or school or child care. Feel free to attach photos or other memorababilia. List the names of schools or daycare facilities attended.

Memories of Grade 1

Record some of your child's friends at home or school or child care. Feel free to attach photos or other memorababilia. List the names of schools, clubs, sporting teams, or daycare facilities.

Memories of Grade 2

Record some of your child's friends at home or school or child care. Feel free to attach photos or other memorababilia. List the names of schools, clubs, sporting teams, or daycare facilities.

Memories of Grade 3

Record some of your child's friends at home or school or child care. Feel free to attach photos or other memorababilia. List the names of schools, clubs, sporting teams, or daycare facilities.

Memories of Grade 4

Record some of your child's friends at home or school or child care. Feel free to attach photos or other memorababilia. List the names of schools, clubs, sporting teams, or daycare facilities.

Memories of Grade 5

Record some of your child's friends at home or school. Feel free to attach photos or other memorabilia. List the names of schools, clubs, sporting teams., or awards.

Memories of Grade 6

Record some of your child's friends at home or school. Feel free to attach photos or other memorababilia. List the names of schools, clubs, sporting teams., or awards.

Memories of Grade 7

Record some of your child's friends at home or school. Feel free to attach photos or other memorabalia. List the names of schools, clubs, sporting teams., or awards.

Memories of Grade 8

Record some of your child's friends at home or school. Feel free to attach photos or other memorababilia. List the names of schools, clubs, sporting teams., or awards.

Memories of Grade 9

Record some of your child's friends at home or school. Feel free to attach photos or other memorababilia. List the names of schools, clubs, sporting teams., or awards.

Memories of Grade 10

Record some of your child's friends at home or school. Feel free to attach photos or other memorababilia. List the names of schools, clubs, sporting teams., or awards.

Memories of Grade 11

Record some of your child's friends at home or school. Feel free to attach photos or other memorababilia. List the names of schools, clubs, sporting teams., or awards.

Memories of Grade 12

Record some of your child's friends at home or school. Feel free to attach photos or other memorababilia. List the names of schools, clubs, sporting teams., or awards.

Memories of Post-Secondary School

Record some of your child's friends at home or school. Feel free to attach photos or other memorabilia. List the names of colleges, universities, tradeschools, clubs, sporting teams., or awards.

Jobs

What was your first job? Record all your jobs on this page. Were they part-time or full-time? How long did you work there?

Observations and Comments

Write down anything you think your child would like to know or read.

Awards and Certificates

Has your child earned a special reward or performed a special act of kindness? Any swimming or skating certificates?